An understanding towards

Irritable Bowel Syndrome

Dedicated to all IBS sufferers
And
Health Professionals

IRRITABLE BOWEL SYNDROME

She stood in the storm and when the wind did not blow her way, she adjusted her sails.

Feel like there are days when you're living on the toilet? Welcome to the world of IBS, a chronic disorder that affects your large intestine triggering symptoms like cramping, abdominal pain, bloating, gas diarrhea/constipation. It is the most common gut disorder worldwide affecting 10-15% of people.

Treatment is not always satisfactory and is done on trial and error basis. It includes: dietary manipulation, low FODMAP diet, medications, psychiatric treatment, hypnotherapy, setting a sleep schedule, exercise, probiotics, yoga and meditation.

A balance of mind-body is important.

The present book looks into all these points and has tried to give answers.

Contents

Page

Forward

I have read through your draft IBS book: most comprehensive and thorough.....well done!
During my complete reading of your book, I have taken the liberty of performing an initial proof read, amending some typographical and sentence-structuring which I hope you will find constructive. This I have done on a printed copy of the document (which is how I work best!) and I will post this to your Boston address.
With respect to a forward to your book, may I suggest the following:

During the last thirty years, working as a busy G.P. in the N.H.S. in England, not a week has passed when I have not been presented with a patient manifesting the symptoms and signs of Irritable Bowel Syndrome (I.B.S.). This condition is ubiquitous and its presentations varied and wide-ranging. The effects of I.B.S. range from the minor and inconveniencing to the severe and life-changing. As with any disease manifesting as a symptom-complex, best treatment will embrace many modalities of intervention.
For many years of my working as a G.P., I had the pleasure of working in association with the author, Dr Pradeep Agarwal, whilst he was employed as a **local** Consultant Colorectal Surgeon and Trust Surgical Director for many years. Dr Agarwal is a technically exceptionally skilled surgeon, widely and expertly trained, and able to produce first-class operative outcomes. However, in my view, what sets him apart from an average surgical approach to a medical problem is his holistic approach to the patient. Nowhere can an all-encompassing patient-centered approach to a problem be more relevant than in the management and treatment of I.B.S.

Dr Agarwal worked in a team which consisted himself, Gastro-intestinal physician, colorectal nurse, a pathologist, a radiologist and a psychiatrist. This was a multidisciplinary approach to look in a particular problem where all aspects were explored. The most common presentation of IBS was abdominal pain. It was commonly presented among young women aged 20-40 years. These patients were referred to him either directly by GPs or Gastro-intestinal physicians. Dr Agarwal consultation with these patients was thorough and investigations and treatment was complete.

In this, Dr Agarwal's second book written since his retirement as an N.H.S. Consultant, Dr. Agarwal explores the many facets of I.B.S. Evidence is investigated and interrogated and mixed with his own professional life-time experiences to formulate a multi-faceted approach to helping the I.B.S. patient, most importantly by achieving an improved understanding of what is a most complex condition. The traditional medical approaches of dietary and medicines interventions are explored but, of greater importance and relevance, Dr. Agarwal critiques and contemplates the so-called alternative routes to management, looking at the role of psychological, physical and life-style interventions as effective and important management strategies.

Dr Agarwal is a spiritual man. His first book written since retirement (An understanding towards Universe and Spirituality) considers the spirit, soul and body speculating upon our very beginnings and origin, life's forces and energies and the concept of God. It is from such a background of contemplation and open thoughtfulness that this diverse piece of work on the subject of I.B.S. derives. As such, this book would be suited to patients and clinicians in all spheres of practice to assist you in achieving an improved understanding of the complexities of I.B.S and I commend this work to you.

Dr Kieron Wiscombe. MB BS, DRCOG, FPCert, DCH.RCP, DOccMed, FRCGP, FIMC.RCSEd

Prologue

I have seen many with IBS symptoms in my clinic crying, and asking for help. They had seen many specialists and received treatment but there was no improvement in their symptoms. I learned from these patients. I reached a conclusion that it is important for the patient to understand his intestinal system and how the digestion of foods may differ in individuals. I also developed an understanding of how important life style is as a contributor to IBS symptoms.

I decided to write a book to provide an understanding towards IBS so that such patients know there is life, perhaps even better, after being diagnosed with IBS. This book is written for those millions of people worldwide who live with all forms of IBS every day. I hope you will find insight into your disease process and hence control of symptoms.

Irritable Bowel Syndrome (IBS) is a collection of symptoms and signs with a specific health related cause. There is a huge problem in our society. IBS has a significant worldwide prevalence. It is estimated that 1 in 6 people in the population suffer from IBS. IBS is associated with disabling symptoms like abdominal bloating, abdominal cramps and pain, diarrhea and constipation. IBS can also severely compromise a person's quality of life.

Many questions arise if one has IBS. What to do about it? What causes it? How to fix my leaky gut? Do I take drugs?

The symptoms could be so severe that your daily routine, as to interfere with activities and professional life curtailed. Imagine having a condition with symptoms so severe that you cannot leave the house, yet your doctor calls it "functional" or "psychosomatic" meaning that it is all in your head!

There are many patients with IBS, some of whom have suffered for decades without relief. Doctors could not find the cause and simply advised to take more fibre or prescribed sedatives, antispam drugs or antidepressants.

There are really only five causes of IBS; allergens, microbes or imbalance of the bugs in your gut, toxins, poor diet and stress. All these can trigger symptoms and create IBS.

Studies have shown that IBS patients have an increased number of outpatient healthcare visits, diagnostic tests and surgical intervention. IBS is associated with a significant healthcare and economic burden to the society.

IBS is often referred to as spastic, nervous or irritable colon. Although the causes of IBS have not fully elucidated, it is believed that symptoms can occur as a result of a combination of factors, including visceral hypersensitivity, altered bowel motility, neurotransmitter imbalance, infection and psychological factors.

It is important for you to get tested for food allergy. You should also test yourself by eliminating foods from your diet which give symptoms, get rid of unwanted bacteria from your gut by taking antibiotic, and repopulate the gut with good bacteria by taking probiotics. Try digestive enzymes with meals to help break down food while your gut heals. You may also benefit from nutrients that help heal the lining of the gut including fish oil, primrose oil, zinc, vitamin A, glutamine and others.

An understanding of your body is very important so that a connection to the mind and body is developed. Non-pharmacological treatment such as dietary modification, exercises, relaxation techniques, meditation and acupuncture are newer modalities to practice.

Re-establishing balance in the autonomic nervous system is an important component of IBS treatment. Behavioral and psychological therapies, stress management also have a role to control IBS symptoms.

Body-mind therapies such as gut-directed hypnotherapy, mindfulness therapy, functional relaxation and body awareness therapy have been used both during treatment and follow-up.

As a Colorectal Surgeon for many years I was referred numerous patients suffering from IBS for years. They were mostly young women where all medical treatment, had failed. The main symptoms were disturbed bowel habit (diarrhea and constipation) and severe abdominal pain. The patients were sent to me to rule out any surgical cause might have been missed. In early time there was not much knowledge in medical field about the pathogenesis, progress and treatment of IBS. There was also lack of technique of imaging of gastrointestinal tract.

Although surgery has no role in treating IBS, the data identify pre-operative misdiagnosis of the aetiology of abdominal pain. This often resulted in abdominopelvic surgery in patients with IBS.

As a Colorectal Surgeon, I was trained to provide surgical and non-surgical treatment for diseases of the colon, rectum and anus. I was able to perform routine screening examinations to reach the diagnosis so that a suitable treatment plan could be established.

Over the years, there has been rapid advancement in the understanding of the aetiology and treatment of IBS. My learning in the disease process also increased and that was reflected in my treating patients differently. The most important aspect of treatment is that patient must develop an insight of his own system. There should be one to one consultation and the patient be encouraged to develop self-confidence.

Although there is much literature available on IBS, there is still a necessity for a book in complete form taking the patient through a journey of his understanding of the disease process. My book covers the entire topic and modern advancement which should be beneficial to both the general public and health professionals.

I have tried to answer some of the relevant points people have asked me over the years.

Introduction

Irritable Bowel Syndrome (IBS) is a long-term condition that affects digestive system. Symptoms of Irritable Bowel Syndrome are sporadic and unpredictable. The most common symptoms include pain or discomfort in the abdomen and a change in bowel habit. The incidence is high and it is thought that about one in ten people in the United Kingdom are affected by this condition. It can develop at any age; the first symptoms often develop at the age between 20 and 30 years. Women are twice likely to get it as men.

At one extreme the symptoms are mild and the person is a healthy individual who does not go to doctor. He does not feel that his life is upset in any way. At the other extreme are those individuals whose life is devastated by IBS. They don't move far from toilet, they feel isolated, panicky and are totally lacking in self-confidence. The social life is ruined and diet is badly restricted. Their tummy becomes the centre of their universe.

Suggestive features are the painful abdominal spasms or stomach cramps, bowel cramps, bloating, constipation and diarrhoea.

The symptoms vary between individuals and affect some people more severely than others. They tend to come and go in periods lasting a few days to a few months at a time, often during times of stress or eating certain foods.

It is common that the symptoms of IBS ease after going to the toilet and opening the bowel.

The symptoms of IBS often improve with lifestyle changes and taking over-the-counter medicines from a chemist. But if symptoms have changed or are new, it's important to consult a doctor.

The condition is often life-long, although it may improve over several years.

The exact cause of IBS is unknown, but most experts think that it's related to increased sensitivity of the gut and problems digesting food. These problems may mean that the person is more sensitive to pain coming from gut. The person may become constipated or have diarrhea because the food passes through the gut too slowly or too quickly.

The symptoms can vary in type, frequency and severity from person to person. However, it is known that stress, illness and diet are significant contributing factors to the condition – and that it can be painful, embarrassing and inconvenient to live with.

IBS occurs when nerves and muscles in the lower bowel aren't functioning as they should, and as a result, the bowel can become much more sensitive to pain.

Most people can trace their IBS back to a period of stress (which can affect the way food is propelled through the digestive system), or to a bout of gastroenteritis "holiday tummy" which may make the intestine overactive and sensitive), or to a course of antibiotics (which may affect the delicate balance of beneficial bacteria in the gut), or to an abdominal/pelvic operation (especially if you had a course of antibiotics beforehand). Whatever triggered it for you, the chances are that stress and some food make it worse.

Please note the following:
- Prolonged periods of stress affect natural digestive rhythm.
- Previous gastrointestinal illness can make bowel more susceptible to IBS.
- Certain foods and drinks can trigger the symptoms of IBS, such as fatty or fried food, processed snacks like crisps or biscuits and drinks that contain caffeine.
- Hormonal changes, such as menstruation, can cause or aggravate IBS.

Please remember that you are not alone; there are countless others experiencing similar challenges with symptoms of IBS.

IBS can be often managed effectively with simple changes to the lifestyle. For example, altering the diet (the diet that works best for you is dependent on your symptoms and how you react to certain foods), taking more exercise (regular exercise, such as light cycling) and altering the fiber in the diet.

IBS symptoms can be reduced by bringing stress levels down, through simple exercise, or relaxation techniques such as meditation.

Digestive System

The human body digestive system is a series of organs that converts food into essential nutrients that are absorbed into the body and eliminates unused waste material. A normal functioning digestive system is essential for good health because if the digestive system shuts down, the body cannot be nourished or rid of waste.

The Digestive System is also known as the gastrointestinal (GI) tract. The digestive system begins at the mouth and includes the oesophagus, stomach, small intestine, large intestine (colon) and rectum. It ends at the anus. The entire system – from mouth to anus – is about 30 feet (9 meters) long.

Mouth   The role of mouth is important to generate saliva (from the salivary glands). Even the smell of food can generate saliva. Saliva contains enzymes, salivary amylase, which breaks down starch. Teeth are a part of the skeletal system and play a key role in digestion. In carnivores, teeth are designed for killing and breakdown meat. In Herbivores, teeth are made for grinding plants and other food to ease them through the digestive process.

Swallowing   Swallowing pushes the chewed food into the oesophagus, where it passes through the oropharynx and hypopharynx. At this point, food takes the form of a small round mass and digestion becomes involuntary. A series of muscular contractions, called peristalsis, transport food through the rest of the system. The oesophagus empties into the stomach.

Stomach and duodenum   The stomach contains gastric juice, which is primarily a mix hydrochloric acid and pepsin, starts breaking proteins and killing potentially harmful bacteria. This process takes an hour or two and then a thick semifluid paste called chyme is formed.
At this point the pyloric sphincter valve opens and chyme enters the duodenum. In the duodenum it mixes with digestive enzymes from pancreas and acidic bile from the gall bladder.

Small intestine   The next stop for the chyme is the small intestine, a 20- foot (6-meter) tube-shaped organ, where the majority of absorption of nutrients occurs. The nutrients move into the bloodstream and are transported to the liver.

The liver creates glycogen from sugars and carbohydrates to give the body energy and converts dietary proteins into new proteins needed by the blood system. The liver also breaks down unwanted chemicals, such as alcohol, which is detoxified and passed from the body as waste.

Large intestine   The leftover material goes into the large intestine (colon). It is 5 feet long (1.5 meters). The primary function of the large intestine is storage and fermentation of indigestible matter.   The large intestine has four parts: ascending colon, transverse colon, descending colon and sigmoid colon. This is where water from the chyme is absorbed back into the body and faeces are formed.
Faeces contains primarily water (75%), dietary fiber and other waste products. Faeces are stored in rectum until they are eliminated from the body through defaecation.

Diseases of the digestive system

Many symptoms can signal problems with GI tract, including: abdominal pain, blood in the stool, bloating, constipation, diarrhoea, heartburn, incontinence and vomiting and difficulty swallowing.

Colon cancer   Among the most widely known diseases of the digestive system is colon cancer. Excluding skin cancers, colon and rectal cancer, or colorectal cancer, is the third most common cancer diagnosed in both men and women.
Polyp growth and formation of irregular cells, which may or may not be cancerous, are the most common development paths for colorectal cancers (also referred to as CRC). These can be detected during a routine colonoscopy. These polyp, if

caught early, can also be removed during colonoscopy, thus eliminating the possibility that they grow further and become cancer.

There are various minimally invasive surgical options available that have good prognosis, for those patients whose cancer has already spread.

It is recommended that asymptomatic patients without a family history begin getting tested (stool, colonoscopy) regularly after the age of 50.

Symptoms which may suggest that colonoscopy is required at an earlier age include rectal bleeding and stool/bowel habit changes which last for more than a few days.

Other diseases

Irritable bowel syndrome (IBS)
Gastro-oesophageal reflux disease (GORD)
Crohn's disease

These diseases can be chronic and are difficult to diagnose and treat.

Food

Many of the diseases of the digestive system are related to the foods we eat, and a number of sufferers can reduce their symptoms by restricting their diets. Many times eliminating acidic things from the diet, such as tomatoes, onions and red wine can have a positive impact.

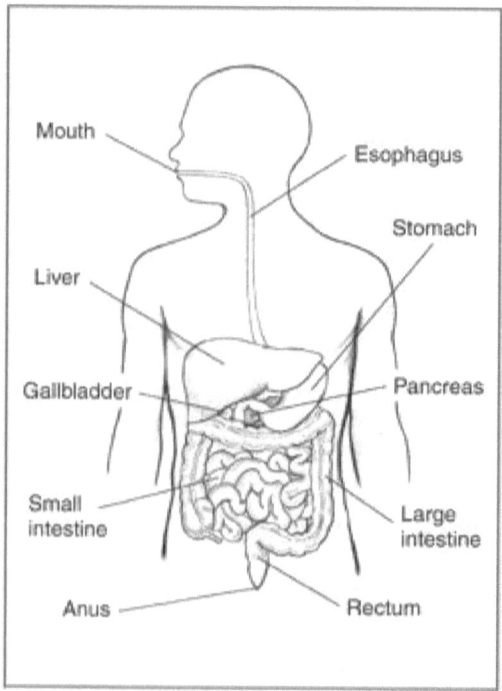

The digestive system

Why is digestion important?

Digestion is important for breaking down food into nutrients, which the body uses for energy, growth, and cell repair. Food and drink must be changed into smaller molecules of nutrients before the blood absorbs them and carries them to cells throughout the body. The body breaks down nutrients from food and drink into carbohydrates, protein, fats, and vitamins.

Carbohydrates. Carbohydrates are the sugars, starches, and fiber found in many foods. Carbohydrates are called simple or complex, depending on their chemical structure. Simple carbohydrates include sugars found naturally in foods such as fruits, vegetables, milk, and milk products, as well as sugars added during food processing. Complex carbohydrates are starches and fiber found in whole-grain breads and cereals, starchy vegetables, and legumes. The *Dietary Guidelines for Americans, 2010,* recommends that 45 to 65 percent of total daily calories come from carbohydrates.[1]

Protein. Foods such as meat, eggs, and beans consist of large molecules of protein that the body digests into smaller molecules called amino acids. The body absorbs amino acids through the small intestine into the blood, which then carries them throughout the body. The *Dietary Guidelines for Americans, 2010,* recommends that 10 to 35 percent of total daily calories come from protein.[1]

Fats. Fat molecules are a rich source of energy for the body and help the body absorb vitamins. Oils, such as corn, canola, olive, safflower, soybean, and sunflower, are examples of healthy fats. Butter, shortening, and snack foods are examples of less healthy fats. During digestion, the body breaks down fat molecules into fatty acids and glycerol. The *Dietary Guide-*

lines for Americans, 2010, recommends that 20 to 35 percent of total daily calories come from fat.[1]

Vitamins. Scientists classify vitamins by the fluid in which they dissolve. Water-soluble vitamins include all the B vitamins and vitamin C. Fat-soluble vitamins include vitamins A, D, E, and K. Each vitamin has a different role in the body's growth and health. The body stores fat-soluble vitamins in the liver and fatty tissues, whereas the body does not easily store water-soluble vitamins and flushes out the extra in the urine.

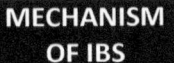
Mechanism of IBS

Pathophysiology of IBS

IBS affects 9%-23% of the world population and more than 10% seek medical attention (1). It is a chronic debilitating functional gastro-intestinal disorder and people affected live a poorer quality of life. The mechanism of the disease is unclear and the complexity and diversity of IBS presentation makes treatment more difficult. The most distressing symptom is abdominal pain and bloating. Other symptoms include diarrhea, constipation, straining at defecation, tiredness and ill feeling.

The mechanism of IBS is complex and incompletely understood. IBS is thought to be multifactorial and both central and peripheral factors are responsible i.e. abnormal GI motility and secretion, visceral hypersensitivity and psychological factors.

The gastrointestinal motor pattern is altered and colonic transit is changed. The gas handling by the gut becomes abnormal and causes bloating. The most important pathophysiological factor is considered the visceral hypersensitivity which causes pain (2).

The visceral pain is characteristic to the IBS and has two of the following three features:
1. Relief by defecation
2. Onset associated with a change in frequency of stool

3. Onset associated with change in the form of stool

IBS affects with the predominance those in the lower socioeconomic groups and 1/3 of the population is affected by it. There are environmental factors involved and IBS seems to be less prevalent with advancing age (3)

Following factors determine the mechanism of IBS:

- Visceral sensitivity
- Abnormal gut motility
- Autonomous nervous system dysfunction

Other important factors developing and influencing the severity of IBS symptoms are:

- Exogenous and endogenous factors   gastrointestinal flora

  Feeding
  Psychological
  factors

- Genetic factors including polymorphisms of human DNA (4)

Visceral Hypersensitivity

The intestine sensitivity is regulated at multiple levels:

- Intestine mucosa and submucosa level
- Spinal cord
- Thalamus

- Cerebral cortex

There are sympathetic (SNS) and parasympathetic (PNS) fibers in the gastrointestinal tract. These are located in the afferent neuron terminals of submucosa (Meissner Plexus) and between the smooth muscle fibers (Auerbach Plexus).

SNS transmits stimuli (Meissner Plexus) which are recognized as abdominal pain at the cerebral cortex level travelling through the thalamus. This pain recognition (afferent fibers) in turn stimulates efferent neural fibers passing through hypothalamus. Efferent neural fibers through PNS (Auerbach Plexus) stimulate or inhibit the contraction of smooth muscle fiber and the secretion of enterocytes (intestinal absorptive cells). These stimuli modify the gut motility and secretion (5).

Visceral sensitivity at enteric mucosa and submucosa

The visceral pain is represented when the mucosa in injured and chemical mediators (ATP, bradykinin) and inflammatory mediators like prostaglandin is released (6). These chemicals directly stimulate afferent fibers at the mucosa (Meissner Plexus) and release histamine, serotonin and 5HT.

During inflammation of the mucosa nerve remodeling can produce chronic hypersensitivity (7) and cascade of the chemical produced exacerbate visceral pain.

There is an increase in nerve contents of the tissue in acute infection which causes an increase in the diameter of nerve fibers.

Visceral sensitivity at spinal cord

Neurotransmitters are released when afferent neurons are triggered (Meissner plexus) by the chemical mediators. This process set up transmission in the synapses between afferent and dorsal horn neurons. A central sensitization is established at the specific pre and postsynaptic receptors (8) and carried up the cerebral cortex via limbic system.

Visceral sensitivity at cerebral cortex and subcortical areas

The visceral pain in IBS is a sharp, aching, or throbbing pain. It is nociceptive pain produced by the injury of the intestinal mucosa. Nociceptive pain is caused by potentially harmful stimuli and is detected by nociceptors around the body. Nociceptors are type of receptors that feel the pain causing harm to the body.
The visceral pain is regulated at the level of thalamus, limbic system and cortex. There are inhibitory neural impulses at the dorsal horn of the spinal cord and this is conducted by GABA neurons (9).
There is an important role of the limbic system situated in brain close to the thalamus and cerebrum. The limbic system supports a variety of functions including emotion, behavior, motivation, long-term memory and smell. There seems to be an interaction between inhibitory pathway and limbic system which is important for the sensation of visceral pain.
There are studies supporting the correlation between IBS visceral hypersensitivity and emotional disorders like depression and bipolar disorders. Abdominal pain can be associated with negative emotional conditions such as fear and grief. More recently in some

new studies, abnormal activities are seen on MRI in cortical and subcortical areas in fearful conditions (10).

Stress is an important factor which modifies the sensation of colon and rectum both in control and IBS patients. The stress induced the release of chemical mediators which in turn stimulate subthalamus receptors (11).

In summing-up, the visceral sensation produced by the stimulation of the colon distension and the substance in the colon and rectum is altered by various mediators at the level of intestinal mucosa, spinal cord, thalamus and cerebral cortex.

Brain-Gut interaction (Autonomous nervous system dysfunction)

There is increasing agreement that autonomic abnormalities can often be associated with functional disorders of the gut.

The visceral hypersensitivity is believed to be the key factor in the mechanism of IBS symptoms. The brain-gut axis interacts at various levels – afferent (ascending) and efferent (descending) pathways, spinal cord, cerebral cortex and subcortical levels.

Psychological factors such as anxiety and depression appear to be important in IBS. There is evidence that gastrointestinal dysfunction also modulates central processes. IBS has also been linked with somatization disorder.

More recently, MRI (magnetic resonance imaging) has played a big role in understanding brain-gut interaction and central dysregulation. Differences in the brain function are noted on MRI in IBS and control. Investigations such as measuring the regional cerebral flow during rectal and colon distention has shown greater activation of certain parts of cerebral cortex and subcortical regions (12). The MRI technique has allowed assessment of the difference in cortical function in response to gut stimulation between healthy control and IBS patients (13). This revelation has permitted potential pharmacologic and behavior intervention.

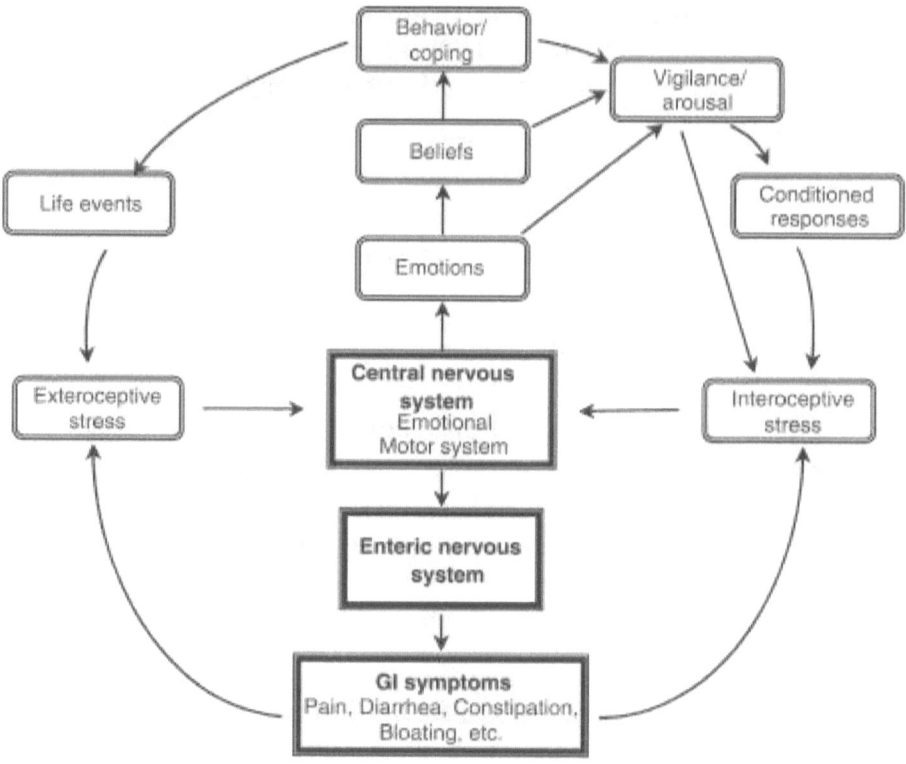

Gut Motility and IBS

Gut motility is the stretching and contractions of gastrointestinal tract (GIT) muscles and it controls movement of food throughout the digestive system. The motility is defined by the movement of the intestine and the transit of the contents within it. When nerves or muscles in any part of the intestine do not function with normal strength and coordination, symptoms related to motility problems develop.

The pattern of the gut contraction can be divided into two categories; peristalsis and segmentation. These come in cycles every 1.5-2 hours but are interrupted by food ingestion. The role of this process is likely to clean excess bacteria and food from digestive system.

Peristalsis occurs soon after a meal. The contractions occur directly behind the bolus of food, forcing it towards the anus into the next relaxed section of smooth muscle. The relaxed section then contracts, moving the bolus of food forward between 2-25 cm per second.

Segmentation also occurs shortly after a meal within a short length of the intestine. In this process longitudinal muscles are relaxed while circular muscles contract. This allows mixing of food and digestive enzymes and a uniform composition is maintained.

Abnormal motility pattern can cause IBS symptoms such as abdominal bloating, pain, nausea, diarrhea and constipation. It is believed that the motor function of the intestine overreacts to stimuli like food and/or stress

As said earlier, nerves in the gut becoming over sensitive to stimuli can also trigger changes in the brain. Symptoms of diarrhea/

constipation are associated with abnormal functioning of autonomous nervous system (sympathetic and parasympathetic).

The colon is the last major organ in the gastrointestinal tract and plays a critical role in regulating the frequency and consistency of stools. Colonic motility dysfunction can cause symptoms like diarrhoea, constipation and intermittent abdominal cramping.

Gastrointestinal flora

The brain-gut axis could be a key factor both in health and disease (14). The brain plays an important role in communicating constantly with the microorganism inside the body (15). The gut-brain axis (GBA) consists of bidirectional communication between the central and enteric nervous system. It establishes a link of emotional and cognitive centres of the brain with the gut functions. Recent advances in researches have described the importance of gut microorganisms influencing these interactions (16)

Bactria are present in the normal gut, especially in in its lower part. They are present in a very high concentration of several billion in the colon.

The normal gut bacterial flora has several important functions:
- They produce substances which has nutritional value
- Protecting against infection by keeping a check on harmful bacteria
- Helping the immune system of the gut to develop

The gut bacteria live in harmony with the body and when this is disturbed disease may occur.

Therapeutic measures may be considered in dealing with the bacteria. Many recent findings suggest that, in part, there may be some dysfunctional interaction between gut flora and the body in causing IBS. This leads to a low-grade inflammation in the gut wall causing IBS symptoms. Therefore, a short-term therapy with antibiotics/probiotics reduces symptoms.

Bacteria communicate with one another through similar electric signaling mechanism as neuron in human brain (17).

King's College London (British Gut) along with American Gut are undertaking a project by collecting data which will tell us how our lifestyle choices and diet influence our microbiome and how we can alter it to reduce disease and other health related problems.

Genes and IBS

More recently researchers have found a mutation of the SCN5A gene which is a subset of IBS. This is a specific genetic defect and causes disruption in bowel function by affecting a sodium channel in gastrointestinal muscles (18).

References

1. Gut Pathogens 2010 2:3

2. Peripheral factors in the pathophysiology of irritable bowel syndrome J. Gunnarsson, M. Simrén Department of Internal Medicine, Sahlgrenska University Hospital, Göteborg, Sweden, Aug 2009

3. Rey E, Talley NJ: Irritable bowel syndrome: Novel views on the epidemiology and potential risk factors. Dig Liver Dis. 2009, 41: 772-780. 10.1016/j.dld.2009.07.005.

4. World J Gastroenterol. 2014 Jun 14; 20(22): 6759-6773

5. Bueno L, Fioramonti J: Visceral perception: inflammatory and non-inflammatory mediators. Gut. 2002, 51 (Suppl 1): i19-23. 10.1136/gut.51.suppl_1.i19.

6. Bueno L, Fioramonti J: Visceral perception: inflammatory and non-inflammatory mediators. Gut. 2002, 51 (Suppl 1): i19-23. 10.1136/gut.51.suppl_1.i19.PubMed CentralView ArticlePubMedGoogle Scholar

7. Millan MJ: The induction of pain: an integrative review. Prog Neurobiol. 1999, 57: 1-164. 10.1016/S0301-0082(98)00048-3.View ArticlePubMedGoogle Scholar

8. Sharkey KA, Coggins PJ, Tetzlaff W, Zwiers H, Bisby MA, Davision JS: Distribution of growth - associated protein,

B-50 (GAP-43) in the mammalian enteric nervous system. Neuroscience. 1990, 38: 13-20. 10.1016/0306-4522(90)90370-J.View ArticlePubMedGoogle Scholar

9. Chen A, Dworkin S, Haug J, Gehrig J: Human pain responsivity in a tonic pain model: psychological determinants. Pain. 1989, 37: 143-160. 10.1016/0304-3959(89)90126-7.View ArticlePubMedGoogle Scholar

10. Price DD: Physiological and neural mechanisms of the affective dimension of pain. Science. 2000, 288: 1769-1772. 10.1126/science.288.5472.1769.View ArticlePubMedGoogle Scholar

11. Talley NJ: 5-hydroxytryptamine agonists and antagonists in the modulation of gastrointestinal motility and sensation: clinical implications. Aliment Pharmacol Ther. 1992, 6: 273-289. 10.1111/j.1365-2036.1992.tb00050.x.View ArticlePubMedGoogle Scholar

12. Naliboff BD, Berman S, Chang L, Derbyshire SW, Suyenobu B, Vogt BA, Mandelkern M, Mayer EA: Sex-related difference in IBS patients: central processing of visceral stimuli. Gastroenterology. 2003, 124: 1738-1747. 10.1016/S0016-5085(03)00400-1.View ArticlePubMedGoogle Scholar

13. Tillisch K, Mayer EA, Labus JS, Stains J, Chang L, Naliboff BD: Sex specific alterations in autonomic function among patients with irritable bowel syndrome. Gut. 2005, 54: 1396-1401.

10.1136/gut.2004.058685.PubMed CentralView ArticlePubMedGoogle Scholar

14. Front. Physiol., 07 December 2011 | https://doi.org/10.3389/fphys.2011.00094

15. IFFGD (International foundation for gastrointestinal disease)

16. Ann Gastroenterol. 2015 Apr-Jun; 28(2): 203–209

17. Biology, Oct 23,2015

18. *Gastroenterology*, 2014; DOI: 10.1053/j.gastro.2014.02.054

Food and IBS

Irritable bowel syndrome (IBS) is an uncomfortable disorder characterized by abdominal pain and dramatic changes in bowel movements varying from diarrhoea and constipation. Abdominal cramps and pain can make everyday activities unbearable. Medical intervention may be necessary to control the symptoms but diet plays an important part in IBS symptoms.

There is a close relationship between the food that people eat and symptoms of IBS they develop. Certain foods trigger diarrhoea and abdominal pain and make symptoms worse. These include eating too much insoluble fibres like skin of fruits and vegetables. Eating chocolates and drinking alcohol, caffeine and drinks rich in fructose or sorbitol can also make IBS symptoms worse.

A healthy diet consists of eating a variety of nutritious foods in moderation. However, certain foods may trigger IBS symptoms. It is important for IBS people to know what foods cause aggravation of symptoms and make a list of them and keep a chart on daily basis.

Symptoms can vary among people so there are no foods on the list to limit or avoid. It is important that IBS people should understand their bodies and tummies to have more regularity, fewer abdominal cramps and less bloating.

List of the foods that can affect IBS symptoms:

1. Insoluble fibers
2. Gluten
3. Dairy
4. Fried food
5. Beans and legumes
6. Caffeinated drinks
7. Processed foods
8. Sugar free sweeteners
9. Chocolate
10. Alcohol
11. Garlic and Onions
12. Broccoli and cauliflower

List of the ways to reduce or eliminate bloating

- Eat less at one time
- Rule out foods intolerant to abdomen by trial and error
- Eat slowly and chew properly so that swallowing air and gases is avoided
- Try foods low in FODMAP and be careful with sugar alcohol

- Avoid being constipated

Insoluble Fibres

Whole grains, vegetables and fruits contain high fibre diet. There are two types of fibres in the food; soluble and insoluble. Soluble fibre attracts water and turns to gel during digestion. This way it slows the digestion. Soluble fibre is found in oat, bran, barley, nuts, seeds, beans, lentils, peas and some fruits and vegetables. It is also found in psyllium (a leafy-stemmed Eurasian plantain, the seeds of which are used as laxative and bulking agent in treatment of IBS and obesity). Insoluble fibre is in whole grains, vegetables and wheat bran. It adds bulk to the stool and helps food pass quickly through the stomach and intestine.

Soluble fibre is good for both diarrhoea and constipation while insoluble fibre is best for constipation only. There are several mechanisms of the dietary fibre acting on the gut: it increases the mechanical stimulation and irritation of the colonic mucosa by increasing the faecal mass and thus causes increased secretion and peristalsis in the intestine. It increases the fermentation by-product in particular to short chain fatty acid (oligosaccharides). These fibers also affect intestinal microbiota, immune system and neuroendocrine system of the gastro-intestinal tract.

Dietary fibre acts on the gastrointestinal tract through several mechanisms, including increased faecal mass with mechanical stimulation/irritation of the colonic mucosa with increasing secretion and peristalsis, and the actions of fermentation by products, particularly short-chain fatty acids, on the intestinal microbiota, immune system and the neuroendocrine system of the gastrointestinal tract (1).

IBS patients should focus on soluble fiber. Insoluble fiber though, may relieve constipation but it can make a person feel bloated.

Fiber rich foods such as fruits, vegetables and whole grains are nutritious and help preventing constipation. However, if you experience bloating from increased fiber intake, try replacing solely to fiber found in fruits and vegetables instead of grains. Following is the list of foods rich in soluble fiber:

1. Grains, like oatmeal and barley
2. Root vegetables, like carrot and parsnips
3. Fruits, like berries, mangoes, oranges and grapefruits
4. Legumes, like peas

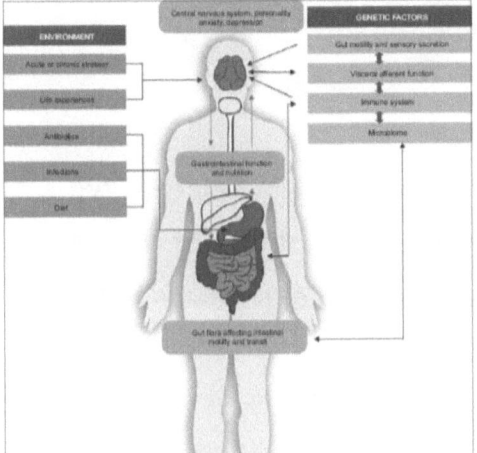

Gluten

Gluten is a kind of protein which is present in rye, wheat and barley. These grains also contain insoluble fires. Some people are allergic to gluten and it can cause symptoms like those of diarrhea-predominant IBS. The condition is called coeliac disease.

Coeliac disease is an autoimmune disorder in which there are changes in the intestinal cells resulting poor absorption of nutrients. These individuals develop reaction to gluten causing ingestion.

In general coeliac disease affects the small intestine while IBS affects the colon.

In some people there is non-coeliac sensitivity where gluten intolerance occurs but without immune response or changes in the intestinal cells. These people may also suffer with the gluten indigestion as those with coeliac disease and have the similar symptoms.

Many people with IBS are also intolerant to gluten and a gluten free diet may improve symptoms. There is test to confirm coeliac disease but there is no such test available to confirm IBS. The recent researches have shown that 4-10% IBS patients also suffer from coeliac disease (2). These patients should benefit from gluten-free diet to improve or eliminate IBS symptoms.

There are more gluten-free products available on shops nowadays like: pizza, cakes, and cookies etc. which are good for people suffering from gluten sensitivity.

IBS patients with no gluten hypersensitivity will continue having symptoms even after eliminating all possible gluten from the diet. These people should look for alternative treatments.

FODMAP

The FODMAP (Fermentable Oligosaccharides, Disaccharides, Monosaccharides and Polyol) diet focuses on reducing or eliminating fermentable, short chain carbohydrates. Foods high on FODMAP are not well absorbed by small intestine and may create more gas and increase fluid in the bowel. This may result in abdominal pain, bloating and diarrhea.

Therefore, Foods rich in FODMAP should be restricted by IBS sufferers. This includes:

- Lactose and dairy
- Products containing high fructose corn syrup
- Added fiber
- Vegetables like broccoli, garlic, onions and artichokes
- Chickpeas and lentils

The foods low on FODMAP, IBS sufferer can enjoy:

- Lactose-free milk and other dairy-free alternatives

- Cheese like feta or brie

- Fruits like kiwi, honeydew melon, cantaloupe and strawberries

- Vegetables like lettuce, carrots, cucumber, bok choy, turnips, potatoes and eggplant

- Proteins like tofu, chicken, fish and egg

It is important to remember that everyone's digestion is different and some IBS can tolerate certain foods, while others may not. It is important to know your body and learn which foods make you feel best. IBS sufferers should limit those foods which do not agree with them react with their intestine.

Diet low in FODMAP should be included in the diet to see if it helps in symptoms. If symptoms improve eat foods low in FODMAP on a regular basis.

Dairy

Dairy may cause IBS like symptoms because of two reasons: firstly it contains fat and secondly it contains a type of sugar called lactose. One can switch to a low-fat or non-fat dairy to lessen the symptoms.

Some people have deficiency of lactase, a type of enzyme necessary to digest lactose in the milk. They suffer from lactose intolerance and have trouble in digesting milk when they eat dairy, like drinking milk, eating cheese or ice cream, yogurt or cheese.

There is no cure for lactose intolerance, but most people are able to control their symptoms by making changes to their diet. These people have a choice for rice milk, almond milk and soy cheese etc.

Casein is primary protein in milk. People who are allergic to milk should avoid milk and all milk products.

Fried foods

Frying actually changes the chemical makeup of the food which affects the gut. High fat contents in fried food can also be blamed for aggravating IBS symptoms.

Deep frying is low cost in food industries and is in high demand. It is widely used because it is acceptable in society and is convenient. In deep frying, high temperature is generated and oil-food interaction takes place. It cooks and dehydrates the food and physical and chemical changes occur. Starch is gelatinized and protein is denatured. The addition of flavouring and colouring also brings changed in the food composition. Some potentially toxic compounds also develop in the oxidised oil (3).

French fries and other fried foods are staple diet of most of the societies in the world. Fried foods are poorly tolerated by IBS patients and they should consider grilling or baking instead frying for a healthier option.

Beans and legumes

Beans in food are very popular and are a near perfect food. They are economic and are high in protein, fibers, vitamins, iron and folic acid. But they can cause IBS symptoms. Beans not only cause constipation by increasing the bulk of stool but can cause bloating and abdominal cramps.

Beans and lentils contain FODMAPs. This is a short chain carbohydrate and sugar alcohol. It is poorly absorbed in the gut and contributes to excessive production of gas causing abdominal pain and bloating. The beans difficult to digest are lima beans, navy beans and soybeans. Easily digestible beans are black-eyed peas, adzuki, anasazi, lentils and mung beans.

The tips to eating beans are: Sort out bad beans, soak the beans overnight or 8+hours, don't stir a lot, pour out soaking water and add fresh water, season by adding with fresh vegetables, like carrot, onion celery and rosemary, do not salt. Cook the beans for an hour or more until tender. Adding cumin (a pinch or two), a bay leaf and 1 inch piece of kombu makes the beans digestible.

Caffeinated drinks

Coffee, soda and energy drinks that contain caffeine can trigger IBS symptoms. Caffeine has stimulating effect on the intestines that can cause diarrhoea. The stimulating effect of caffeinated drinks increases the gut motility aggravating IBS symptoms.

Some observational studies have shown 26-40% people have aggravation of their IBS symptoms after drinking caffeinated products (4). The symptoms recur when caffeine is reintroduced after been stopped (5). Adding milk or cream in coffee may also contribute towards IBS symptoms.

Other effects of caffeine on the gut are: elevation of stress hormones (cortisol, epinephrine and norepinephrine), the acidity of caffeine irritates the intestine, caffeine speeding up the gastric emptying, decreased absorption of magnesium caused by caffeine which irritates colonic mucosa causing diarrhoea.

IBS patients therefore are advised to restrict their caffeine intake.
There are options worth trying by trial and error. Such as: reduce coffee intake, choose a different brand, try decaffeinated, switch to tea, try dairy alternatives, and change the sweetener.
If caffeine triggers IBS symptoms seriously then consider eliminating it altogether.

Processed Foods

Processed foods often contain additives and preservatives that might flare IBS symptoms. The common food additives are: monosodium Glutamate (MSG), Artificial Sweeteners (Aspartame and Saccharine), BHT (Butylated Hydroxytoluene), BHA (Butylated Hydroxyanisole), Carrageenan, High Fructose Corn Syrup (HFCS), Trans Fats and Sodium Nitrates.

MSG is a common additive and is used to intensify the flavour of savoury dishes, frozen dinners, salty snacks and canned soups. It is also added in restaurants and fast food places. MSG consumption is also associated with weight gain. Some people are sensitive to MSG and experience IBS symptoms and headaches.

Trans fats are associated with inflammation and intestinal symptoms which makes up as much as 60% of total fats in these products. Carrageenan is found to cause IBS symptoms and intestinal ulcers in animal studies. High-fructose corn syrup contributes high calories in diet and is associated with weight gain, diabetes and abdominal cramps.

Sodium nitrate is a common ingredient in the procced food that is converted into harmful compound called nitrosamine. It is high risk in several cancers and can make IBS symptoms worse. In addition other additives; thickeners, emulsifiers, colourants as well as plastic and contaminants released by high temperature heating may play IBS symptoms worse.

It is found that IBS patients consume fewer vegetable than their healthy counterparts.

Steamed Frozen Vegetables

Steamed vegetables are a healthy option for those who want to increase their vegetable intake. They are not only still rich in fiber they are rich in insoluble fibers. This gives a feeling of fullness which helps in limiting calories. While fresh fruits and vegetables should be the first choice, steamed vegetables are a healthy choice and promotes healthy digestive system.

Boiling vegetables may deplete some of the nutrient contents from the food such as folic acid and vitamin C. Steaming vege-tables requires less time and water and so nutrients are lost at its minimum.

Sugar free sweeteners

The commercial sweeteners are also referred as sugar alcohols, polyols, artificial sweeteners and sugar substitutes. They are used in sugarless candy, gum, most diet drinks and some mouthwash. These products contain ingredients like sucralose, acesulfame, potassium and aspartame. These substances are hard to digest and make IBS symptoms worse.

IBS patients should avoid all sugar-free drinks made with artificial sweeteners containing polyols. These include sweeteners ending in "-ol" such as sorbital, mannitol, maltitol and Xylitol, also isomalt. These are found in diet sodas, sugar-free juices and sugar free teas.

Some IBS patients are intolerant to fructose. They should avoid juices high in fructose such as, mangos, pears, apples and watermelon.

What to drink?

Enjoy as many foods and drinks as you can tolerate but eliminate the offenders. Drinks which are easily tolerated by IBS patients are as following:

- Fruit juices   cranberries, bananas, grapefruits, lemons, grapes and pineapples.
- Vegetable juices   carrots, celery, chives, broccoli, cucumber, ginger, parsley, pumpkin, spinach, tomato, turnips squash
- Herbal tea   that does not contain caffeine
- Ginger drinks
- Dairy free milkRice milk, soy milk, oat milk, almond milk etc.

Pay attention to the response of your body to different drinks.

Alcohol

Alcohol can increase the severity of IBS symptoms. Alcohol and IBS are not a good combination. Alcoholic beverages are toxic and can trigger IBS symptoms because the way the body digests alcohol.

Alcohol is shown to irritate the gut flaring up the IBS symptoms. Even a small amount of alcohol drink is enough to trigger IBS symptoms and cause cramping and bloating. The severity of symptoms including diarrhoea depends upon the sensitivity of an individual to alcohol. Wines and mixed drinks usually contain sugar and beer contains gluten.

The recommendation for IBS patients is:

- Avoid carbonated beverages that adds air and gas into the tummy
- Avoid sweet mixes, juice and sugary cocktail that contain FODMAPs which are easily fermented sugar and triggers up the IBS symptoms.

Alcohol can also be dehydrating and can affect the liver function and digestion.

Chocolates

Chocolates have high concentration of caffeine and high sugar content and can trigger IBS symptoms. However, specifically dark chocolate also contains antioxidants that may help lowering blood pressure and improve circulation.

Chocolates were thought to be gut irritant but the new science reveals some health benefit of chocolates. The dried seed that makes chocolates contains flavanol which has positive cardiovascular and neurological effects on the body. It may lower blood pressure, help reversing insulin resistance, decrease blood cholesterol and slows age related memory decline.

According to the new researches, coca may serve as a prebiotic and encourages healthy balance of gut bacteria. Very little of cocoa flavanol is absorbed in small intestine. It is passed on into the colon and interacts with bacteria in the colon (7,8,9). In one study consumption of a drink rich in cocoa flavanol over a four weeks period changed beneficial gut bacteria and bifidobacteria and lactobacillus were increased. The disease causing bacteria were inhibited preventing diseases caused by such bacteria (7,8,9).

It is also found that most commonly used prebiotics e.g. fructooligosaccharides and galactooligosaccharides are high in FODMAPs. These do not necessarily increase the level of lactobacillus microbes. This new information makes cocoa a potentially a prebiotic option for IBS patients (7,8,9).

The higher the percentage of cocoa in chocolate, the healthier it is. Darker chocolate contains more cocoa. Cocoa can be added into smoothies. Following is the list of chocolates one can eat, provided one's tummy allows:

- Dark chocolate: 15-20 Gram.
- Milk and white chocolate: 15 Grams if not lactose intolerant
- Cocoa powder: 2-4 heap teaspoons
- Drinking Chocolate (23-60%): less than 35 Grams

Chocolates can cause constipation which increases IBS symptoms.

Spicy foods

Spicy foods can aggravate abdominal pain and IBS symptoms. A greater number of specific nerve fibers were found in the colon of IBS patients that reacts to a substance within chili powder.

Abdominal pain is common in IBS patients. The capsaicin receptor TRPV1 (transient receptor potential vanilloid type 1) may play an important role in visceral pain. TRPV1 – immunoreactive nerve fibres were investigated in colonic biopsies from IBS patients, and this was related to abdominal pain (10).

Garlic and Onion

Garlic and onions are used to flavour the food, but they can be difficult to digest. They can produce gas causing abdominal cramps and bloating triggering IBS symptoms.

The use of garlic and onion is forbidden to people practicing yoga. Onions and garlic constricts the vibrational channels (nadis) preventing a person from experiencing mental clarity and higher states of consciousness.

There was once a debate in 2007 in the center of Roma at La Trattoria restaurant where the chief chef Filippo La Mantia stopped using garlic on the basis that it a stinky ingredient and overpowers the delicate flavour of food prepared. The acceptability of garlic and onion by the gut depends how much sulphur your colon can handle, friendly bacteria in your colon, how much raw or cooked garlic is consumed and types of spices and vegetables are used. As any sulphur rich ingredient, onions and garlic are very heating, although cooking destroys much of the sulphur.

Onions and garlic also have some good effects which have been highlighted in the media. Such as: lowering high blood pressure, reduce high cholesterol, they are natural antibiotics, anti-fungal and antibacterial and are blood cleanser. They also increase sperm count.

Unfortunately, onions and garlic do have negative effects on the body and the gut. Onions and garlic produce a chemical called allicin (2-propene-1-sulfinothioic acid S-2-propenyl ester) which is responsible for their strong pungency and aroma.

All alliums produce sulphur molecules, is easily dispersible in the air and attack nose and eyes. Chopping and eating opinion and garlic stink.

Garlic is a powerful herb and traditionally used in Ayurvedic medicines, but is not recommended in food for daily consumption. Garlic, as a broad spectrum antibiotic kills not only the bad germs but also the most needed friendly germs and thus changes the colonic bacteria environment. This is the reason IBS symptoms may be aggravated after consumption of onions and garlic.

Onions and garlic develop Rajo and Thamo Gunas and hence a person is unable to achieve sense control that is important to reach to the Krishna Consciousness.

Are people in India becoming addicted to onions and garlic? Once a national party in India was defeated because of very high price of onions and garlic. So, people got so angry and changed the government. This is because of the attachment towards the food which has many negative effects on the body.

Broccoli and cauliflower

Certain vegetable cause gas and abnormal bowel habits such as Cruciferous vegetables: broccoli, cauliflower, cabbage, cole-slaw, sauerkraut, artichoke, brussels, onions, shallots, leeks and asparagus.

Broccoli and cauliflower are difficult to break down in intestine and are difficult to digest. They produce gas and can cause constipation and thus trigger IBS symptoms.

Grating broccoli and cauliflower might make the digestive process simpler for the intestine but won't eliminate IBS symptoms.

These vegetables have high level of sulphur which mixes up with the chemical in the stomach, like acid and forms hydrogen sulphide. This leads to gas formation with a foul smell.

Is IBS linked to the genes?

In a recent genome-wide study, IBS is found to have an association to certain DNA variants in only women. It can explain why the condition is less common in men (11).

Genetic factors were suspected but were poorly studied. In the study an increased risk for IBS was found to be significantly associated with genetic variants on chromosome 9 in women (chromosome 9q31.2).

References

1. Dietary Fibre in irritable bowel syndrome **Magdy El-Salhy,[1,2,3] Synne Otterasen Ystad,[3] Tarek Maz-zawi,[2,3] and Doris Gundersen Int J Mol Med. 2017Sep: 40(3): 607–613. Published online 2017 Jul 19. doi: 10.3892/ijmm.2017.3072**

2. Gluten vs. Irritable Bowel Syndrome (IBS) -

    https://www.verywellhealth.com/gluten-vs-irritable-bowel-syndrome-562696

3. *Keliani Bordin, Mariana Tomihe Kunitake, Keila Kazue Aracava, Carmen Silvia Favaro Trindade:* Archivos Latino Americano De Nutricion

    Volumen 63, No 1, Ano 2013

4. Simren, M., et al., Food-related gastrointestinal symptoms in the irritable bowel syndrome.Digestion, 2001. 63(2): p. 108-15.

5. Nanda, R., et al., Food intolerance and the irritable bowel syndrome. Gut, 1989. 30(8): p. 1099-104

6. Brown, S.R., P.A. Cann, and N.W. Read, Effect of coffee on distal colon function. Gut, 1990. 31(4): p. 450-3.

7. Brickman, A., et.al. "Enhancing dentate gyrus function with dietary flavanols improves cognition in older adults." *Nature Neuroscience* 2014 17:1798-1803.

8   Corti, R., et.al. "Cocoa and Cardiovascular Health" *Circulation* 2009 119:1433-1441.

9   Monash University Low FODMAP Diet App Accessed May 26, 2015.

10 A Akbar, P Facer, JRF Walters, P Anand, S Ghosh: Increased capsaicin receptor TRPV1-expressing sensory fibres in irritable bowel syndrome and their correlation with abdominal pain, Neurogastroenterology, volume 57, issue 7

11 IBS linked to genetic variant found only in women: Bonfiglio F, et al. *Gastroenterol.* 2018;doi:10.1053/j.gastro.2018.03.064.April 9, 2018

Gut and immune system

Irritable bowel syndrome (IBS) is a functional disorder; the pathogenesis is poorly understood. IBS is associated with abdominal pain and alteration of bowel habit. The symptoms greatly impair the person's quality of life. It has put intense economic burden on the community.

There are some evidence of low-grade inflammation and innate immune system dysfunction in the development of the disease process. Mast cells (MC), eosinophils and other key immune cells together with their mediators seem to play an important role. There seems to be cytokine imbalance in the intestinal mucosa and systemic circulation.

IBS was regarded as an exclusively functional disorder, but recent studies have shown evidence of low-grade mucosal inflammation in some IBS patients. There are several mechanisms which can explain the pathogenesis of IBS: post-infectious alternations (1), dysfunctional epithelial permeability (2), abnormalities in gut microbiota (3) and elevated stress level (4) can enhance or stimulate immune response. A combination of low-grade inflammation of the intestinal mucosa with impaired bowel motility and visceral sensitivity could explain the underlying etiology and pathology of IBS.

Some studies have shown overlapping pathways between IBS and inflammatory bowel disease (IBD), such as dysregulated immune activation and abnormalities of the enteric system (5, 6).

Post-infectious irritable bowel syndrome

Post-infectious IBS is observed in patients following a bout of infectious gastroenteritis (7); the incidence is seen is about 10% reported cases (8). The mechanism of this is poorly defined, but may include genetic factors, cytokine production and host bacteria interaction as well as molecules involved in controlling mucosal permeability (tight junctions) (9).

IBS-like symptoms develop in about 50% of patients with microscopic colitis (10) and 33-57% of patients with ulcerative colitis or Crohn's disease in remission (11, 12). These figures are substantially higher than the expected prevalence of IBS in general population. This supports the view of ongoing low grade mucosal inflammation in IBS patients.

The gut and immune system are closely linked together. In fact 70-80% of the body immune system is situated the digestive tract. The digestive system is responsible for a person's overall well-being. In order to achieve this, good bacteria in the gut, specialized immune cells and hormones work together to keep the Gastro-intestinal tract at its optimum level (13).

There are approximately 500 different bacteria in the gut living. The weight of these bacteria is about two to three pounds. One of the most important functions of commensals bacteria is boosting the immune system. They produce antibiotics that fight harmful viruses and bacteria.

The digestive system is responsible for overall well-being. In order to achieve it is important to keep the GI tract at its optimum level. In order to do this, the good bacteria in the gut, specialized immune cells and hormones work together.

The nervous system may affect the immune system via direct innervation of immune organs and by secretion of hormones from pituitary and other endocrine organs. The nervous system regulates the speed at which food moves through the digestive tract.

There are various routes for pathogens to breach the first line of defense of the body, the digestive system being a major one. The food and drink we consume can easily be contaminated with bacteria and viruses. Our stomach plays a crucial role in killing many of these off. Further down the digestive system, the gut wall forms a gastrointestinal barrier. However, in some cases this barrier may be violated. If

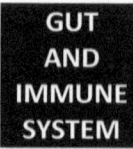
pathogens enter the circulation, the immune system takes action to defend the body.

The inside cell lining of the gut wall are usually packed tightly together forming a barrier to prevent the pathogens entering the gut wall. In IBS the tight junctions of the cell lining is broken creating gaps through which the bacteria enter the gut wall. It is called "leaky gut". In IBS irritation of the gut wall, together with muscles spasm (often with diarrhea) pathogens enter the gut wall and cause inflammation. In case of constipation, the waste product moves slowly in a leaky gut. This results toxins compromising the immune system even more.

In IBS it is possible that bacterial or yeast overgrowth is residing in the gut. The normal pathogens multiply and become detrimental.

Is IBS an Autoimmune Disorder?

IBS is not an autoimmune disorder; it is a functional bowel disorder. However, some autoimmune disorders mimic or overlap with IBS. For example, coeliac disease and inflammatory bowel disease (IBD) cause similar symptoms as IBS and must be ruled out when making a diagnosis of IBS (14). There is some confusion between a functional disorder and immune system abnormalities in at least one type of IBS – called post-infectious IBS.

What is an autoimmune disorder – and how it is different from IBS?

Normally the immune system defends the body against harmful bacteria, viruses, toxins etc. In case of autoimmune disorder the body is incapable differentiate between an invader and his own normal tissue. In autoimmune disorder, the person's immune system mistakenly attacks his own healthy body tissue (15).

IBS is classified a functional bowel disorder, which means that there is a problem in signaling connection between the gut and brain. Therefore, the digestive system does not function properly but there is no structural problem present (16). While autoimmune diseases can be detected with blood and imaging tests, there are no such tests for functional disorder such as IBS.

Healthy ways to strengthen the immune system

1. Don't smoke.
2. Eat a diet high in fruits and vegetables.
3. Exercise regularly.
4. Maintain a healthy weight.

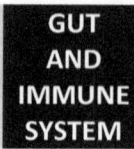

5. If you drink alcohol, drink only in moderation.
6. Get adequate sleep.
7. Take steps to avoid infection, such as washing your hands frequently and cooking meats thoroughly.

References

1. Spiller R, Garsed K. Postinfectious irritable bowel syndrome. Gastroenterology. 2009;136:1979–1988.[PubMed]

2. Piche T, Barbara G, Aubert P, et al. Impaired intestinal barrier integrity in the colon of patients with irritable bowel syndrome: involvement of soluble mediators. Gut. 2009;58:196–201. [PubMed]

3. Simrén M, Barbara G, Flint HJ, et al. Rome Foundation Committee. Intestinal microbiota in functional bowel disorders: a Rome foundation report. Gut. 2013;62:159–176. [PMC free article] [PubMed]

4. Qin HY, Cheng CW, Tang XD, Bian ZX. Impact of psychological stress on irritable bowel syndrome. World J Gastroenterol. 2014;20:14126–14131. [PMC free article] [PubMed]

5. Spiller R, Major G. IBS and IBD - separate entities or on a spectrum? Nat Rev Gastroenterol Hepatol. 2016;13:613–621. [PubMed]

6. Scanu AM, Bull TJ, Cannas S, et al. *Mycobacterium avium*subspecies paratuberculosis infection in cases of irritable bowel syndrome and comparison with Crohn's disease and Johne's disease: common neural and immune pathogenicities. J Clin Microbiol. 2007;45:3883–3890. [PMC free article] [PubMed]

7. Spiller R, Garsed K. Postinfectious irritable bowel syndrome. Gastroenterology. 2009;136:1979–1988.[PubMed]

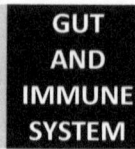
8. Thabane M, Kottachchi DT, Marshall JK. Systematic review and meta-analysis: The incidence and prognosis of post-infectious irritable bowel syndrome. Aliment Pharmacol Ther. 2007;26:535–544.[PubMed]

9. Dunlop SP, Jenkins D, Neal KR, Spiller RC. Relative importance of enterochromaffin cell hyperplasia, anxiety, and depression in postinfectious IBS. Gastroenterology. 2003;125:1651–1659. [PubMed]

10. Barbara G, Stanghellini V, Cremon C, et al. Aminosalicylates and other anti-inflammatory compounds for irritable bowel syndrome. Dig Dis. 2009;27(suppl 1):115–121. [PubMed]

11. Spiller R, Garsed K. Postinfectious irritable bowel syndrome. Gastroenterology. 2009;136:1979–1988.[PubMed]

12. Thabane M, Kottachchi DT, Marshall JK. Systematic review and meta-analysis: The incidence and prognosis of post-infectious irritable bowel syndrome. Aliment Pharmacol Ther. 2007;26:535–544.[PubMed]

13. https://www.health24.com/.../your-gut-is-the-cornerstone-of-your-immune-system-20...

14.Lacy BE, Chey WD, Lembo AJ. New and emerging treatment options for irritable bowel syndrome. Gastroenterol Hepatol (N Y). 2015;11(4 Suppl 2):1-19.

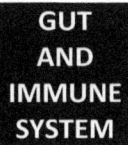
15.MedlinePlus. Autoimmune disorders. Accessed July 20, 2016 at: https://medlineplus.gov/ency/article/000816.htm.

16.International Foundation for Functional Gastrointestinal Disorders. Functional GI Disorders. Accessed 7/14/16 at: http://www.iffgd.org/gi-disorders/functional-gi-disorders.html.

Treatment of IBS

IBS is an incurable condition. It is a common long term, sometimes lifelong, problem of the intestine. It is characterised by recurrent abdominal pain, bloating and constipation or diarrhoea predominant symptoms.

The common age for IBS symptoms to start is 20-30 years but it can develop at any age of life. It is thought to affect 1 in 5 people at sometimes of life.

The exact cause of IBS is not very clear, but most experts think that IBS is related to increased sensitivity of the gut and problems digesting food. A person becomes constipated or has diarrhoea because the transit time (speed of the food passing through the gut) is either too slow or too fast. The stress in life also plays an important part in aggravating IBS symptoms.

Treatment is mainly symptom-based and the essential part of treatment is making changes to diet and lifestyle.

The key factors of the treatment are as following

- Know your body and tummy
- Identify and avoid foods and drinks that aggravate symptoms
- Alter the amount and type of fibre in diet
- Exercise regularly
- Stay calm, control emotions and stress level

- Medication, hypnotherapy, psychotherapy, acupressure and acupuncture are sometimes prescribed to the individual symptoms experienced

In controlling IBS symptoms it is important to understand the nature of the condition. Changing diet and lifestyle are first steps towards getting relief from the symptoms.

IBS diet

There is no single diet which fits to all. It all depends what food a person reacts to. Therefore, it is necessary to know your daily pattern, food you eat and symptoms you get. It is recommended to keep a food diary to identify foods which do not agree with your system and trigger IBS symptoms. The foods do not agree with your body should be avoided or eliminated.

Fibres

There are two types of fibres in food: Insoluble and soluble. Insoluble fibres do not dissolve in water and soluble fibres dissolve in water. Foods rich in insoluble fibres are: wholegrain bread, bran, cereals, nuts and seeds (not linseeds). Food rich in soluble fibres are: oat, barley, rye, fruit (banana and apple), root vegetables (carrots and potatoes) and golden linseeds.

If you have diarrhoea then one must cut down on the insoluble fibres, that means avoid skin, pith and pips from fruits and

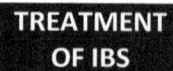

vegetables. In case of constipation, increase the amount of soluble fibres and water in your diet.

Diet Low in FODMAP (fermentable oligosaccharides, disaccharides, monosaccharides and polyols)

These are the carbohydrates which are not easily digestible and are not broken down for absorption by the gut. Therefore, they start to ferment in the gut quickly. During the process gas is released which can lead to bloating.

Low FODMAP diet could be effective in controlling bloating. It means avoiding or eliminating foods high in FODMAP such as animal milk, wheat and beans products and certain fruits and vegetable. It may be necessary to consult a dietician to understand the low FODMAP diet.

General guidelines for IBS patients on what to eat:

- Eating meals at a regular time. Do not rush Chew the food properly and take time to eat
- Do not miss meals or eating after a long gap
- Drinking at least eight cups of fluid a day in particular water. Non-caffeinated drinks such as herbal tea can also be considered
- Alcohol and fizzy drinks should be avoided
- Caffeinated drinks, tea, coffee should be avoided
- Consider sticking to low FODMAP foods. It will avoid eating resistant starch that is not digested in small intestine

and reaches the colon in intact form. The resistant starch is often found in processed foods and the foods which are re-cooked

- Fruits should be consumed in limited way to three portions a day

- In diarrhoea predominant IBS, eliminate sorbitol (an artificial sweetener) found in sugar free sweets, chew gum and drinks and slimming diets.

- Eat oats (cereal, porridge) and linseeds if you have excessive flatulence and bloating.

Exercise and IBS

Exercise is a part of behavioral modification of change of life style and helps in controlling IBS symptoms. Exercise also reduces stress which is a well-known factor and contributes triggering IBS symptoms. Nerves in the colon controls contraction of colon muscles which help propelling food in a coordinated fashion. Stress, however, affects these nerves which cause abdominal pain and constipation.

IBS can also results in weight gain or loss in certain individuals. Exercise is helpful in these situations. Exercise is important for two main reasons: firstly, it relieves stress and secondly, it makes the gut function better. The sluggish body makes the gut slower. An active and fit body makes the gut regular and healthier.

It is important that exercise is done as a daily prescription. Exercise taken for 20-30 minutes three to five times a week can make improvement in IBS symptoms. Walking for 30 minutes daily is also considered relieving IBS symptoms (1).

Important steps before starting exercise are:

- Exercise should be done at the time when the intestine is quieter

- Avoid eating two hours before. The best time is in mornings when the intestine is also quieter

- Caffeine or hot drinks have speeding effects on the bowel contraction. These drinks are better avoided before setting up exercise

- Fatty and gas-producing foods should be avoided prior to the exercise.

- Try to exercise each day at the same time

- Choose an exercise that fits in with your way of life

Intensity of exercise varies from person to person. In case of diarrhoea predominant IBS the body may not cope with intense exercise such as running, fast walking, running, swimming, cycling etc. for a prolonged period. In this situation try to cut back and observe if IBS symptoms improve. In case of 10 minutes a mile running, cut it back to 12-13 minutes and see if that makes any improvement. Sometimes jerky movements on the body while running, irritates the gut. Walking is a good alternative in this situation.

Exercise can reduce stress and constipation that is a common occurrence in people with IBS. It also improves heart and lung functions. Exercise in general improves wellbeing and improves overall magnitude of IBS symptoms.

Reducing stress and psychological treatment

Psychological stress is an important factor for development of IBS. More and more clinical and experimental evidence showed that IBS is a combination of irritable bowel and irritable brain. People with IBS frequently suffer from anxiety and depression, which can aggravate symptoms.

It is important to learn that there are diverse factors in the development of IBS. These include: psychological stress, intestinal infection, intestinal immune system disruption and/or inflammation, changes in the intestinal microbiota or bacterial overgrowth and genetic transmission. Abuse and early life learning have also been found to contribute to the development of IBS syndrome (2,3). Psychological stresses have marked impact on intestinal sensitivity, motility, secretion and permeability.

There is strong evidence that IBS is a stress sensitive disorder. Therefore, the treatment of IBS should pay attention to managing stress and stress induced responses. These include: patient-physician relationship, patient education, hypnotherapy, cognitive behavioural therapy, dietary modification, dietary modification, exercise, biofeedback therapy (4).

There is an emerging concept of a microbiota-gut-brain axis. Chronic evidence induces dysbiosis (a term for a microbial imbalance and impaired microbiota) which may contribute to several diseases including IBS (5). Intestine is a natural reservoir of microbiota and plays a physiological role in metabolic, protective and structural functions in the body. This gives an approach towards targeting microbiota to treat IBS (6). Pharmacological drugs treating gastrointestinal and psychological symptoms should be used to treat irritable bowel and irritable brain.

The role of 5-HT is well known in stress related disorders, such as anxiety, depression and chronic pain syndrome. 5-HT also plays a critical role in altering gut motility, visceral sensitivity and intestinal secretion (7). 5-HT4 receptor antagonists were investigated and were found to relieve some symptoms of IBS (8). Strategies targeting serotonin systems have also been investigated in treating IBS (9).

Following activities can reduce the stress level significantly:

- Relaxation techniques- 　meditation, breathing exercises

- Physical activities - 　Yoga, pilates, tai chi

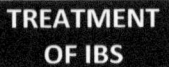

- Regular exercise -   walking, runni8ng,
  swimming

Stress counselling or cognitive behavioural therapy (CBT) could also be beneficial in reducing the stress level.

Medication

Medication can also be helpful in relieving IBS symptoms. These include:

- Antispasmodics   These are helpful in reducing abdominal pain and

                         cramps

- Laxatives   These are helpful in relieving constipation

- Antimotility medicines These are helpful in relieving diarrhoea

- Low dose antidepressants These are helpful in reducing abdominal pain

                         Independent of antide-
                         pressant effect

Abdominal pain is caused by contraction of smooth muscles of the intestine. Antispasmodics are used to relax smooth muscles and help in reducing abdominal pain. Smooth muscles are within the wall of hollow organs and circle the intestine. The intestine and colon are squeezed when smooth muscles contract causing pain. These muscles are involuntary and are under direct control of unconscious part of the brain.

A number of different medications can be used to help treat IBS, including:

- Antispasmodics – which help reduce abdominal (stomach) pain and cramping.

    Antispasmodics work by relaxing muscles in digestive system such as mebeverine and peppermint oil in therapeutic doses.

- Laxatives – which can help relieve constipation. Bulk-forming laxatives are recommended in people with IBS. They make stool softer that are easier to pass. It is important to drink plenty of water while using a bulk forming laxative.

- Antimotility medicines – which can help relieve diarrhoea. These medications slow down the contraction of muscles in the bowel and so the speed of the food passing through the intestine slows down. This allows more time for the stool to harden and solidify.

    Lopermide is usually recommended in IBS patients.

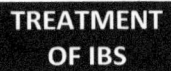

- Low-dose antidepressants – which were originally designed to treat depression but can also help in reducing stomach pain and cramping independent of any antidepressant effect.

  There are two types of antidepressant are used to treat IBS: tricyclic antidepressants (TCAs) and selective serotonin reuptake inhibitors (SSRIs). They are helpful in controlling pain and cramping by preventing signals being sent to and from the nerves in digestive system.

  Example of TCAs is amitriptyline and SSEIs citalopram.

- Newer drugs

  Eluxadoline.   Eluxadoline is an oral agent with mixed opioid effects (μ- and κ-opioid agonist and δ-opioid receptor antagonist) twice-daily doses of 75 mg and 100 mg (10)

  Peppermint oil. A new sustained-release formulation of peppermint oil has recently demonstrated efficacy in IBS (11)

  Bile acid sequestrants. Increased appreciation for the contribution of bile acid malabsorption to IBS-D symptoms raises the possibility that some patients may benefit from therapy with bile acid sequestrants. (12)

Medication should be used according to the symptoms and type of IBS you suffer from

There are four types of diabetes:

- Constipation predominant (IBS-C)

- Diarrhoea predominant (IBS-D)

- Mixed, alternate constipation and diarrhoea (IBM-M)
- Unsubscribed, symptoms do not fit in above categories, abdominal pain and bloating (IBS-U)

Medication should be used in consultation with the doctor according to the IBS symptoms.

Constipation

- Polyethylene glycol (PEG)
- Linaclotide (Linzess)
- Lubiprostone (Amitiza)
- Plecanatide (Trulance)
- Loperamide (Imodium)
- Bile acid sequestrants (cholesterol lowering medicines)

Diarrhoea and abdominal pain

- Alosetron (Lotronex)
- Eluxadoline (Viberzi)

Following drugs are helpful in conjunction with others

- Bulking agents such as psyllium
- Antibiotics such as rifampicin

Abdominal pain and bloating

- Antispasmodics
- Antidepressants

- Probiotics

Pain medications

- Pregabalin (Lyrica)
- Gabapentin (Neurotin)

Probiotics

Probiotics are dietary supplements that contain "friendly bacteria" (especially those with a predominance of Bifidobacterium infantis) and these may help in improving digestive health. Probiotics are supposed to establish a natural balance of the gut bacteria when it has been disrupted.

Some IBS patients find taking probiotics help in relieving symptoms; however, there is little evidence to support this.

Probiotic can make IBS symptoms worse if FOPMAP sugar is used as a base in making it.

Psychological treatments

The cause of IBS is poorly understood. There are various reasons described in the pathogenesis of IBS. There are two main reasons:

- Alteration of muscle contraction of the bowel
- Increased sensitivity of the bowel mucosa to the distension and movement of food, gas or faecal material through the gut.

Other factors aggravating IBS symptoms are:

- Eating, stress and emotional arousal
- Gastrointestinal infection
- Menstrual period
- Gaseous distension

Do these psychological and increased negative moods contribute triggering IBS symptoms? Are IBS symptoms a result of many years of disrupted life activities?

There are several different types of psychological therapies. All these teach the techniques to control IBS symptoms.

- Psychotherapy - This technique involves talking to a trained psychotherapist to look deeper into the problems and worries.
- Cognitive behavioural therapy (CBT) - This is a type of psychotherapy that involves examination how beliefs and thoughts are linked to the behaviour and feelings. This technique teaches ways to alter behaviour and thinking to cope with the situation.
- Hypnotherapy - In this technique hypnosis is used to change the unconscious mind's attitude towards the symptoms.

Complementary therapies

These include as following:

- Aqua pressure and acupuncture
- Reflexology
- Meditation
- Mindfulness training -   This is the act which makes the person aware of their senses and feelings at every moment, without interpretation or judgment.

Special Medications for IBS

- Alosetron (Lotronex)   Alosetron relaxes the colon and slows the waste moving through. It is can only be prescribed by doctors enrolled in special program. It is indicated in IBS women suffering from severe diarrhoea-predominant symptoms.
- Eluxadoline (Viberzi)   Eluxadoline can ease diarrhoea by reducing bowel muscles contraction and fluid secretion in the intestine.
- Rifaximin (Xifaxan)   This antibiotic can decrease bacterial overgrowth and diarrhoea.
- Lubiprostone (Amitiza)   Lubiprostone can increase fluid secretion of the small intestine helping with the passage of stool. It is approved for women with constipation-predominant symptoms.
- Linaclotide (Linzess)   This can also increase fluid secretion in small intestine to help passing stool.

Potential future treatments

- Serum-derived bovine immunoglobulin/protein isolate (SBI)
  This could be helpful in diarrhoea-predominant IBS.
- Enteric-coated peppermint oil   These are specially coated tablets that slowly release peppermint oil in small bowel.   They ease bloating, urgency and abdominal pain and pain while passing stool.

Vitamin D and IBS

Vitamin deficiency was found in about 80% of IBS patients. The reason of this is poorly understood but this condition should be treated.

Antihistamines and IBS

Histamine in the body s released during allergic reaction. It is also released by the gut due to the allergens when food is passing through causing inflammation. A trial of antihistamines (Loratidine or Cetirizine) could be beneficial to IBS patients.

Gut Microbiota and IBS

The microbial ecosystem in the gut must be healthy to keep a person healthy. The imbalance of gut bacteria can make a person sick. It is estimated that there are 500 species (about three pounds) of bacteria in the gut. There are good and bad bacteria. There is more bacterial DNA than human DNA in a person's body.

IBS is caused mainly by two reasons: food allergy and overgrowth of bacteria in the bowel. But there could be other causes such as lack of digestive enzymes, parasites living in the gut, zinc or magnesium deficiency, heavy metal toxicity etc.

Bacterial overgrowth is a syndrome that can be treated by a 10 days course of Rifaximin and can result improving bloating and other IBS symptoms.

Small bowl overgrowth can be diagnosed by a breath test which measure gas production by bacteria or by urine test that measures by-products of bacteria after they are absorbed into the system.

Setting a sleep schedule

The body clock is governed by the biological clock and so are the gut functions. Melatonin supplement at bed time regulate the body clock and can be helpful when travelling across time zones.

References

1. Endurance Sports Nutrition (2007) Eberle, S.G. Human Kinetics.

2. Camilleri M, Di Lorenzo C. Brain-gut axis: from basic understanding to treatment of IBS and related disorders. J Pediatr Gastroenterol Nutr. 2012;54:446–453. [PMC free article] [PubMed]

3. Sperber AD, Drossman DA. Irritable bowel syndrome: a multidimensional disorder cannot be understood or treated from a unidimensional perspective. Therapy Adv Gastroenterol. 2012;5:387–393.[PMC free article] [PubMed]

4. Halland M, Talley NJ. New treatments for IBS. Nat Rev Gastroenterol Hepatol. 2013;10:13–23.[PubMed]

5. Bonfrate L, Tack J, Grattagliano I, Cuomo R, Portincasa P. Microbiota in health and irritable bowel syndrome: current knowledge, perspectives and therapeutic options. Scand J Gastroenterol. 2013;48:995–1009. [PubMed]

6. Cryan JF, Dinan TG. Mind-altering microorganisms: the impact of the gut microbiota on brain and behaviour. Nat Rev Neurosci. 2012;13:701–712. [PubMed]

7. Christine N. Yohn, Mark M. Gergues, and Benjamin Adam Samuels: The role of 5-HT receptors in depression, Mol Brain. 2017; 10: 28

8. Houghton LA[1], Jackson NA, Whorwell PJ, Cooper SM 5-HT4 receptor antagonism in irritable bowel syndrome: effect of SB-207266-A on rectal sensitivity and small bowel transit. Aliment Pharmacol Ther. 1999 Nov;13(11):1437-44.

9. Mohammad Fayyaz and Jeffrey M Lackner Serotonin receptor modulators in the treatment of irritable bowel syndromeTher Clin Risk Manag. 2008 Feb; 4(1): 41–48., Published online 2008 Feb.

10. 64. Lembo AJ, Lacy BE, Zuckerman MJ, et al. Eluxadoline for irritable bowel syndrome with diarrhea. N Engl J Med. 2016;374(3):242–253. [PubMed]

11. 65. Cash BD, Epstein MS, Shah SM. A novel delivery system of peppermint oil is an effective therapy for irritable bowel syndrome symptoms. Dig Dis Sci. 2016;61(2):560–571. [PMC free article] [PubMed]

12. Stotzer PO, Abrahamsson H, Bajor A, Sadik R. Effect of cholestyramine on gastrointestinal transit in patients with idiopathic bile acid diarrhea: a prospective, open-label study. Neuroenterology. 2013;2:1–5. doi: 10.4303/ne/235657. [CrossRef]

Psychiatric treatment and IBS

IBS is a functional bowel syndrome and is associated with a poor quality of life. IBS is reported to occur more frequently in women than men. The most common age is between 20 and 40 and the female to male ratio is 2:1. It is speculated that sex hormones may alter the regulatory mechanism of the brain-gut-microbiota axis in the pathophysiology of IBS (1).

It is a painful condition and is associated with significant psychological distress and higher level of anxiety and depression. It puts a negative impact on quality of life (2). The gut motility and visceral hypersensitivity are affected by the changes in emotional state.

There is a direct communication between brain and the bowel. In IBS there is dysfunction in the central nervous system, or in the bowel or a combination of both (3). Changes are noted in prefrontal lobe, cerebral cortex and thalamus on neuroimaging studies indicating that the part of the brain is altered which deals with attention, emotion and pain modulation (4).

The main aim of the treatment of IBS and its related symptoms is to improve the quality of life. In the most circumstances, doctors treat IBS with traditional medicines. However, these medicines are ineffective or temporarily relieve IBS symptoms. People are trying to understand the background of IBS problem and are looking for alternative treatments. The association between the brain and the bowel is well established. Psychiatric treatments are proposed which mind/body treatment includes hypnotherapy, cognitive behavioural therapy and psychodynamic therapy. The concept is based on the acceptance of one's own state and focus on the changing awareness.

There is a major role of mind/body dysfunction in the development of IBS but other peripheral changes such as altered bowl motility, visceral hypersensitivity and bacterial overgrowth should not be ignored. The mind/body model will be appropriate to understand the development, maintenance and treatment of IBS symptoms (5,6).

There is clinical evidence that visceral hypersensitivity is enhanced in presence of stress (7).

Treatment Themes of IBS derived from mind/body relation

GI symptoms-specific anxiety (meal related events, abdominal pain or diarrhoea) is characterised by increased fear and worry about GI sensation (sometimes even mild ones) and increased attention to them (vigilance). Another part of GI symptoms is avoidance of any situation that might be associated with symptoms and a strong desire to limit oneself to a safe place and activities.

The mind/body psychologic therapies are based on the following understandings (8):

- Stress can stimulate colon spasms, resulting is abdominal discomfort. The stressful life is associated with increase visceral activity.
- IBS patients coping response to the bowel activities is poor and inappropriate. They are constantly aware towards their visceral sensations.
- IBS patients have low self-esteem and suffer from depression. There is psychological fear, social withdrawal and isolation.
- IBS can pressurise relationships, marriages, friendships and employment. It can affect the sex life.

Psychological Treatments

In general psychological treatments are reserved for patients with moderate to severe symptoms, in particular if they experience psychological distress.

Treatments used

- Psychotherapy   dynamic and cognitive-behaviroal therapy
- Relaxation therapy
- Hypnotherapy
- Biofeedback therapy
- Mindfulness-based therapy

The choice of treatment depends on the patient requirement, available resources and experience of the therapist. Psychological treatments can also be combined. It is important to understand the background of stress in each individual patient.

Cognitive behavioural therapy

CBT helps patients change their habitual thoughts, feelings and behaviour that may magnify stress responses and negative moods by applying a series of self-exploration exercises and stress reducing strategies.

CBT was first developed to treat depression. Patients build insight into the relationship between each of the factors (thoughts, behaviour, physical reaction and emotions) and learn ways to intervene thoughts, their behaviour and their physiologic responses to improve mood and emotions. For example, patients may learn to identify and change unhelpful thinking pattern and change in relaxation exercises; similarly changing behaviour (avoidance and isolation) that may contribute to physical or psychological distress.

CBT is the most widely- study psychotherapy for IBS. CBT focuses on the following components:
1. Psychoeducation about the stress response and its relationship
2. Building insight into cognitive and behavioural responses to IBS symptoms and/or fear of symptoms
3. Modifying their responses to decrease distress related to IBS and decrease physical reactivity to stress.

CBT can be delivered effectively in groups, telehealth or internet-based protocols (9). For less motivated patients face to face format may be preferred.

Relaxation therapy

The stress response is "flight or fight" phenomena.   In IBS the body demands to sit up and pay attention.

Relaxation techniques are excellent techniques to gain control on a stressful situation. The techniques include visualisation, deep breathing and progressive muscle relaxation.

Visualisation   It is important to educate yourself and identify the situations triggering IBS symptoms. Find a comfortable chair and spend 10 minutes, twice a day practising new skills. First thing is to visualise yourself in a calm, peaceful and relaxing place. By focusing on such a place, attention is diverted away from worrisome thoughts. This way positive and active step is taken which will help in coping and manage IBS symptoms better.

Deep breathing and progressive muscle relaxation   create a body experience that is the exact opposite of what is needed in time of stress. This relays a different message to the brain, a message of safety, which allows the brain to "stand down" and diminish the stress response.

Progressive relaxation of muscles

1. The first step is to take a deep breath and flex stomach muscles (by sucking the stomach) as much as possible for five seconds.
2. Then exhale, letting all tension out of the muscles.
3. Repeat as comfortable.

Different techniques work for different people. Be sure to have patience with yourself as learning these skills takes time.

Hypnosis

Hypnosis is the induction of consciousness in which a person apparently loses the power of voluntary action and is highly responsive to suggestion or direction. Hypnosis uses relaxation techniques and self-suggestion to help patients gain a more positive feeling about their IBS symptoms. These treatments are targeted in large part to symptom-specific problems such as fears and coping.

During this process, a clinician helps the client into a particular psychological state involving both highly-focused attention and deepened relaxation. Once in this state, the clinical teaches the client how to gain control of physiologic responses and symptoms that are not usually under conscious control.

Hypnosis for IBS involves progressive relaxation, and then suggestions of soothing imagery and sensations focused on the individual's symptom.

A study has demonstrated that the beneficial effects of hypnotherapy are long lasting for up to five years. There is also a continued improvement in symptoms, thus giving patients better control over their condition (10).

A potential criticism for the use of hypnotherapy in treating IBS is expensive because of the time a therapist spends. However, there is sustained effect, efficacy and control of IBS symptoms in majority of patients. This offset the cost of treatment by reducing the cost of medication and other healthcare demands.

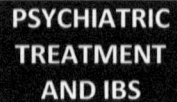
Biofeedback therapy

Biofeedback is a process that enables an individual to learn how to change physiological activity for the purposes of improving health and performance. Biofeedback sessions include real-time monitoring of an individual's physiological signals which are then displayed back to the individual. The goal of biofeedback is to use this feedback to help the individual develop self-awareness of their physiological states. This awareness may lead to a better control over autonomic activity and improved health outcomes.

Mindfulness based therapy

Mindfulness is an awareness of a situation in a conscious mind. Mindfulness therapeutic technique involves achieving a mental state by focusing one's awareness on the present moment, while calmly acknowledging and accepting one's feelings, thoughts and bodily sensations.

Mindfulness is the basic human ability to be fully present, aware of where we are and what we're doing, and not overly reactive or overwhelmed by what's going on around us.

Mindfulness based strategies supported the benefits in controlling IBS symptoms is some studies (11).

References

1. Mulak A, Taché Y, Larauche M. Sex hormones in the modulation of irritable bowel syndrome. World J Gastroenterol. 2014;20:2433–2448. doi: 10.3748/wjg.v20.i10.2433. [PMC free article] [PubMed][Cross Ref]

2. Stasi C, Bellini M, Bassotti G, Blandizzi C, Milani S. Tech Coloproctol. 2014. Serotonin receptors and their role in the pathophysiology and therapy of irritable bowel syndrome. [PubMed]

3. Mayer EA, Tillisch K. The brain-gut axis in abdominal pain syndromes. Annu Rev Med. 2011;62:381–936. doi: 10.1146/annurev-med-012309-103958. [PMC free article] [PubMed] [Cross Ref]

4. 20. Piché M, Chen JI, Roy M, Poitras P, Bouin M, Rainville P. Thicker posterior insula is associated with disease duration in women with irritable bowel syndrome (IBS) whereas thicker orbitofrontal cortex predicts reduced pain inhibition in both IBS patients and controls. J Pain. 2013;14:1217–1226. doi: 10.1016/j.jpain.2013.05.009. [PubMed] [Cross Ref]

5. Drossman DA. Presidential address: Gastrointestinal illness and the biopsychosocial model. Psychosom Med. 1998;60:258–67. [PubMed]

6. Naliboff BD, Munakata J, Chang L, Mayer EA. Toward a biobehavioral model of visceral hypersensitivity in irritable bowel syndrome. J Psychosom Res. 1998;45:485–92. [PubMed]

7. Mayer EA, Craske MG, Naliboff BD. Depression, anxiety and the gastrointestinal system. J Clin Psychiatry. 2001;62:28–36. [PubMed]

8. Bruce D. Naliboff, Michael P. Fresé, and Lobsang Rapgay . Evid Based Complement Alternat Med. 2008 Mar; 5(1): 41–50. Published online 2007 May 17. doi: 10.1093/ecam/nem046

9. Moss-Morris R, McAlpine L, Didsbury LP et al. A randomized controlled trial of a cognitive behavioural therapy-based self-management intervention for irritable bowel syndrome in primary care. Psychol Med 2010; 40: 85–94. [PubMed]

10. W M Gonsalkorale, V Miller, A Afzal.   Long term benefits of Hypnotherapy for IBS. Gut. 2003 Nov;52(11);1623-1629

11. Ljótsson B[1], Andréewitch S, Hedman E, Rück C, Andersson G, Lindefors N. Exposure and mindfulness based therapy for irritable bowel syndrome--an open pilot study. J Behav Ther Exp Psychiatry. 2010 Sep;41(3):185-90. doi10.1016/j.jbtep.2010.01.001. Epub 2010 Jan 7.

Acupuncture and IBS

Acupuncture is a system of complementary medicine in which fine needles are inserted in the skin at specific points along what are considered to be lines of energy (meridians), used in the treatment of various physical and mental conditions.

Acupuncture is a popular alternative therapy for IBS. According to researchers at the national Institutes of Health (NIH), acupuncture is proven effective for treating chronic pain and abdominal bloating.

There is consistent evidence that a course of acupuncture improves IBS symptoms and general wellbeing though there are arguments about the extent to which the effect is placebo-related. Researches have shown that acupuncture treatment may benefit IBS symptoms by:

- Providing pain relief

- Regulating the motility of digestive tract

- Raising the sensory threshold of the gut. Various possible mechanisms have been identified, involving spinal nerves and NMDA receptors (N-methyl-D-aspartate receptors) and a range of neurotransmitters. A lowered threshold to bowel pain and distension are hallmarks of IBS.

- Increasing parasympathetic tone. Stress activates the sympathetic nervous system, which can stimulate colon spasms, resulting in abdominal discomfort. In IBS people, the colon can be oversensitive to the smallest amount of conflict or stress. Acupuncture activates the opposite parasympathetic nervous system, which initiates the relaxation or "rest and digest" response.

- Reducing anxiety and depression. The distress provoked by IBS symptoms can lead a vicious cycle of anxiety-pain-anxiety, while the embarrassing nature of the condition can lead to feelings of depression. Acupuncture can alter the brain's mood chemistry, increases production of serotonin and endorphins, helping to combat these negative affective states (1,2)

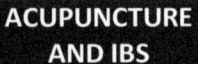

Acupuncture can be safely and effectively combined with other treatments, relaxation exercises, herbal medicines and psychotherapy.

Acupressure

This is one of the potent reflexology pressure points used in treatment of IBS and digestive disorders. This acupressure point is located halfway between the lower end of the breastbone and the belly button (naval).

References

Akehurst R, Kaltenthaler E. Treatment of irritable bowel syndrome: a review of randomised controlled trials. Gut. 2001 Feb;48(2):272-82.

Maxwell PR et al. Irritable bowel syndrome. Lancet. 1997 Dec 6;350(9092):1691-5.

Yoga, meditation, Spiritualism and IBS

Yoga is an old discipline from India. It is both spiritual and physical. Yoga uses breathing techniques, exercises and meditation. It helps to improve health and happiness.

The main goal of Yoga is achieving physical and mental health. Yoga in daily life teaches to achieve good health, inner peace and harmony.

Yoga helps in controlling mind, body and soul. It brings together physical and mental disciplines to achieve a peaceful body and mind. It helps managing stress and anxiety and keeps a person relaxed. It also helps increasing flexibility, muscle strength and body tone.

Yoga builds muscles and can reduce fat by burning calories. It increases heart rate which aids up boosting metabolism. A regular Yoga can play a big role in controlling weight. Certain Yoga postures can make the abdomen stronger and flatter. The twisting and bending movements in Yoga may also help in reducing bloating.

Meditation is about training in awareness and getting a healthy sense of perceptive. It is learning to observe your own thoughts and feelings without judgement so that eventually a better insight is developed. It is training the mind to the subconscious and possibly the unconscious level. It will help for better understanding to your own feelings and emotions. By learning about deeper states of consciousness, one can open his subconscious mind and create his reality at will and with precision. It is important to understand different brain frequencies:

1. Beta (14-40 Hz) reasoning wave

   The waking consciousness and

2. Alpha (7.5-14 Hz)

   The deep relaxation wave

3. Theta (4-7.5 Hz) wave

   The light meditation and sleeping

4. Delta (0.5-4 Hz)

   The deep sleep wave

5. Gamma (above 40 Hz)   The insight wave

   This range is most recently discovered and is fastest frequency at above 40 Hz. Gamma waves are associated with burst of insight and high-level information processing.

   The gamma wave is a pattern of neural oscillation in humans with frequency between 25 and 100 Hz though 40 Hz is typical. Gamma waves may be implicated in creating the unity of conscious perception (the binding problem) (1).

A simple meditation is using the transition from Beta or Alpha to Theta state by focusing on the breath. The breath and mind work in tandem, so as breath begins to length, brain waves begin to slow down. In doing meditation; one should sit comfortably in chair or on the floor with crossed-legs and shoulders relaxed, spine tall.

Learning to meditate is like learning any other skill. It takes consistent practice to get comfortable. It is important to understand how the brain contributes to the state of mind. The subconscious mind plays a big role in fulfillment and establishes co-ordination between the body, mind and soul.

Mindfulness is the ability to be present; to rest in the here and now, fully engaged with whatever we're doing in the moment.

For many health care providers the treatment of IBS is more problematic than the diagnosis. Firstly, the patient's symptoms should be determined in terms of severity. Mild symptoms are occasional in nature and daily activities are not interfered. Moderate symptoms are more frequent and have some impact on daily activities (such as home life, social activities, professional life). Severe symptoms are present on daily basis and have a significant impact on daily activities (2).

It is estimated that at least 40% of health care professionals use some form of alternative therapy in treating their patients. This number is thought to be even higher in patients with functional gastrointestinal disorders (3).

The effect of stress on the development and expression of IBS symptoms is well established. Many patients worldwide practice Yoga to improve their overall health. The discipline of Yoga means to attain unity with mind, body and spirituality. It has been practiced for thousands of years and is an integral part of Ayurveda (traditional Indian medicine).

The current hypothesis of the basis behind Yoga is the reduction of stress and alternation of the brain-gut interaction, improved sleep, improved quality of life, changes in autonomic system function and possibly changes the gut microbiome.

The most common techniques focus on body posture (Asnas), breathing (Pranayama), or meditation (Dhyna).

In some studies Yoga practiced on a regular basis, may be as effective for a young woman as a walking program at improving IBS symptoms (4). The emphasis should be given on precisely aligned postures and the physical intensity a few times a week can modulate the stress and affect the brain-gut axis. The Yoga appears to be generally safe. It provides some respite from busy work schedule or home.

However, it is not possible to make a firm recommendation about the use of yoga for the treatment of IBS.

Advantages of yoga can be summarized as following:

- Reconnect with your body
- Manage stress and anxiety
- Increase blood flow and circulation
- Balance your hormones
- Process challenging emotions

References

1. Ian Gold (1999). "Does 40-Hz oscillation play a role in visual consciousness?". *Consciousness and Cognition.* **8** (2): 186–195. doi:10.1006/ccog.1999.0399. PMID 10448001.

2. Drossman DA, Chang L, Bellamy N, et al. Severity in irritable bowel syndrome: a Rome Foundation Working Team report. Am J Gastroenterol 2011;106:1749–1759.

3. Barnes PM, Bloom B, Nahin RL. Complementary and alternative medicine use among adults and children: United States, 2007. Natl Health Stat Report 2008;1–23.

4. Shahabi L, Naliboff BD, Shapiro D. Self-regulation evaluation of therapeutic yoga and walking for patients with irritable bowel syndrome: a pilot study. Psychol Health Med 2016;21:176–188.

IBS and Herbs

At times, it can be challenging to control IBS symptoms. It is useful to learn some of the herbal remedies thought to be good for the digestive system. It is important to talk to your doctor before trying herbal remedies. These herbs are thought to improve overall digestive health.

Peppermint Oil

Peppermint oil is the only herbal supplement which could be effective in reducing abdominal pain. It is the only herbal medicine approved by the American College of Gastroenterology for its quality (1,2).

Peppermint oil appears to relax the gut muscles and reduces muscle spasms that contribute to abdominal pain. However, the overuse of peppermint oil can cause nausea, diarrhoea, vomiting and abdominal pain as well.

Slippery Elm

Slippery elm is known to Native Americans and is used as a remedy for a variety of health conditions. It calms down mucosal irritation by coating the lining of the intestine.

It adds the bulk to stool and is used in IBS symptoms of pain, diarrhoea and constipation (3).

Artichoke Leaf Extract

This newer remedy is also used to reduce IBS symptoms effectively. In a meta-analysis artichoke has reduced bowel frequency to regulate bowel movement (4).

Aloe Vera

It is also effective in controlling IBS symptoms.

Herbs for constipation

There are several herbal preparations effective in treating IBS constipation. They are as following:

Amalaki   This is a fruit of the Amalaki tree and is found throughout Asia. It is often used in Ayurvedic medicine. It has a positive effect in digestion and is used as a laxative.

Triphala   It is a herbal preparation made of three fruits; bibhataki, haritaki and amalaki. In addition to being a laxative it reduces abdominal pain and bloating.

Herbal stimulant laxatives   These contain anthraquinones and are used as stimulant laxatives. These include senna, cascara, rhubarb and frangula.

Herbs for diarrhoea

There are herbs which may be useful in diarrhea-predominant IBS.

Chamomile   It is thought to reduce gut inflammation and reduces intestinal spasm. It is available in tea, liquid and capsule form.

Berry leaf teas   It contains tannins which reduces intestinal inflammation and secretion. It includes blueberry, blackberry and raspberry leaves.

References

1. Ford AC, Moayyedi P, Lacy BE, et al. American College of Gastroenterology Monograph on the Management of Irritable Bowel Syndrome and Chronic Idiopathic Constipation. *Am J Gastroenterol*. 2014;109(SUPPL. 1):S2-S26. doi:10.1038/ajg.2014.187.

2. Ford AC, Moayyedi P, Chey WD, et al. American College of Gastroenterology Monograph on the Management of Irritable Bowel Syndrome. *Am J Gastroenterol*. 2018:S1-S18. doi:10.1038/s41395-018-0084-x.

3. Bundy R, Walker AF, Middleton RW, Marakis G, Booth JC: Artichoke leaf extract reduces symptoms of IBS and improves quality of life. J. Altern Complement Med. 2004 Aug; 10(4); 667-9

4. Hamid Reza Bahrami, Shokouhsadat Hamadi, Roshnak Salari, Mohammadreza Noras: Herbal Medicines for Management of IBS: A systemic review. Electronic Physician 2016 Aug; 8 (8): 2719-2725

Epilogue

Remember your IBS does not define you; your strength and courage does. A contributing factor to IBS symptoms is when you eat and how much you eat in one sitting. Modern lifestyle is busy and snacking is the most treacherous of all. It is important to eat slowly and chew well. Spread out your meals throughout the day and do not skip a meal. An early evening meal around 6-7 pm is beneficial.

It is important to connect your mind to your body and know your body as a whole. Eliminate relevant dietary components to get rid of common food sensitivities and foods that do not agree with you. Try to avoid dairy, gluten and sugar and try eating simple diet for two to three weeks.

An elimination diet involves removing foods from your diet that you suspect your body can't tolerate well. The foods are later reintroduced, one at a time, while you look for symptoms that show reaction. It takes 5-6 weeks to identify foods contributing to your symptoms.

It is useful to keep a diary for a few months of what you eat or drink, the time and outcome. Change your eating and drinking habits. Eat small amounts over the day and chew well. Drink a lot of water.

IBS is a functional bowel disorder and presents with functional abdominal bloating, functional constipation, functional diarrhoea, bloating and abdominal pain. There is a complete lack of evidence of organic disease however, it is important to consult your doctor regularly to exclude the presence of some other pathology.

The unpredictability of IBS makes people suffer and dignity may be lost. Healthcare personnel should allow patients to talk about their suffering and discomfort.

Abdominal bloating could be predominant symptom in IBS. Bloating occurs because of excess of gas in the intestine. There are many possible causes of bloating; from overeating to air swallowing, constipation, hormone fluctuation, food allergies and IBS. Some of the common foods which cause bloating are greasy, fried foods, and foods with high sodium content causing water retention. There are some typical "gassy" vegetables, such as broccoli, cauliflower and legumes such as beans.

Following are tips to avoid too much bloating:
- Eat slowly and chew well (this prevents you from swallowing too much air)
- Avoid artificial sweetener and low fat choices containing it

- Avoid regular chew hum (it causes air to swallow)
- Avoid drinking too much coffee
- Develop an awareness of foods to which you have intolerance
- Don't eat when you are not hungry

Be aware of lactose intolerance which is found in milk and dairy products. Fructose intolerance is intolerance to the sugar found in fruits, honey and some commercial products. Overgrowth of bacteria in the small intestine is common in IBS patients. Consult your doctor.

Some other useful tips:

- Peppermint essential oil: Rub a small amount into your hands with body lotion. Massage in circles on your stomach. Always allow an hour after eating before trying this.
- Try probiotics
- Try herbs. Try Candibactin BR two capsules three time a day for a month for bacterial overgrowth; BS Candibactin AR two capsules three times a day for yeast overgrowth.
- Vitamin A, Zinc, Omega-3 fats (fish oil) evening primrose oil and glutamine may be helpful.
- Try herbs like quercetin and turmeric to reduce inflammation and leaky gut

Following complimentary treatment could be beneficial in some individuals:

- Acupressure and acupuncture
- Yoga and meditation
- Regular whole body and abdominal exercises

Acknowledgement

I would like to thank my wife and son for their constant encouragement in writing this book. My wife had come across patients suffering from IBS symptoms who had consulted various doctors but with little relief. The symptoms were so intense that their lives became meaningless at home, work and socially. My wife constantly searched for a solution and encouraged me to write on this frequently talked about subject.

Although, there is a lot of literature available on IBS, it lacks the clarity and completeness. The lack of understanding of the behaviour and lack of evidence to the disease process has made people and health professionals confused.

I have been a Colorectal Consultant Surgeon for many years and worked in NHS and private sectors. My fellow colleagues at work and in my social life have provided me with extraordinary support. I worked closely with Dr. Martin Fairman, a retired Gastro-intestinal physician. He has thoroughly reviewed this manuscript to be useful to both general public and health professionals.

My thanks go to Dr Kieron Wiscombe and his wife Sarah for their extraordinary professional support. Kieron is a retired GP and Sarah a retired advanced Nurse Practitioner. Their presence and constant feedback of the patients' progress has been immensely helpful in writing the book.

I am grateful to the time of Bunny helping in formatting and publication of the book.